KARBVELOUS KETO

Transform your Plate, Transform Your Life
Thanksgiving Edition

Carolyn Boheler, PhD

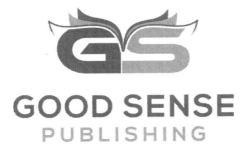

GOOD SENSE
PUBLISHING

Introduction to Karbvelous Keto-Thanksgiving Edition

Thanksgiving is a holiday steeped in tradition, family, and a generous dose of indulgence. For many, the holiday conjures up images of golden turkey, creamy mashed potatoes, warm rolls, and a lineup of desserts that makes any sweet tooth sing. But for those of us who have embraced the Keto lifestyle, Thanksgiving can feel like navigating a minefield of hidden carbs and sugar-laden temptations. It's a challenge I know all too well, having spent many years adjusting my lifestyle to not only manage my health but also find a way to thrive and celebrate.

In this Thanksgiving edition of *Karbvelous Keto*, I'm here to help you transform the holiday plate into something that's both satisfying and aligned with your health goals. Each recipe has been crafted to keep you on track without compromising the essence of traditional flavors. Think of it as the best of both worlds—a Thanksgiving that's rich in flavor but light on carbs, honoring both our cravings and our commitment to a healthier lifestyle.

This book offers a curated collection of classic Thanksgiving dishes, revamped for a Keto-friendly table. Here, you'll find all the elements of a memorable meal: appetizers to keep everyone happily snacking while the turkey finishes roasting, main courses with hearty, savory flavors, side dishes that give a low-carb twist to beloved classics, and desserts that will end your meal on a sweet, guilt-free note.

Thanksgiving is more than just a meal—it's a chance to connect, celebrate, and savor life's blessings. Let's make this holiday one to remember, not just for its flavors, but for how good you'll feel staying true to your health journey.

I am not a medical doctor, and nothing in this book should be taken as medical advice. It's essential to consult with your own doctor before beginning any diet or lifestyle change to ensure it's safe and suitable for you. My background is not in the medical field; my doctorate is in metaphysics and religion. This book is intended to offer insights and ideas based on my personal experience and research but should never replace professional medical guidance.

I've included links to items found on Amazon that are used in the recipes within this book. When you click one of these links, I may earn a small commission, but rest assured, your price will not be higher because of it. Occasionally, you might even find a better deal!

The links are clickable on the kindle or ebook versions, or you can find a page of links at www.GoodSensePublishing.

Tips and Tricks For Enjoying a Keto Thanksgiving

Sticking to Keto during Thanksgiving doesn't mean you have to miss out on the flavors and joy of the holiday. With a little planning and a few smart strategies, you can savor a Thanksgiving meal that's satisfying, flavorful, and completely Keto-compliant. Here are some tips to help you enjoy every bite of the holiday feast without derailing your Keto goals:

Plan your Plate: Start with Protein

- The star of most Thanksgiving tables, the turkey, is naturally Keto-friendly. Start your plate with a hearty serving of turkey, focusing on the skinless breast or dark meat if you prefer extra flavor. This helps you fill up on protein and fats, which are essential for staying satisfied and energized on Keto.

Make Sides that Shine without the Carbs

- Traditional sides like stuffing, mashed potatoes, and rolls are typically high in carbs, but Keto offers delicious alternatives. Think about cauliflower mash instead of potatoes, stuffing made with low-carb bread or veggies, and roasted Brussels sprouts with crispy bacon. By having these options ready, you'll be less tempted by carb-heavy dishes.

Bring a Keto Dish To Share

- If you're celebrating with family or friends, bring a Keto-friendly dish or two to the table. This way, you know you'll have options you can enjoy without worry. Plus, it's a great way to introduce others to delicious, healthy alternatives that still taste incredible.

Go Heavy on Herbs and Spices

- The magic of Thanksgiving lies in its flavors—sage, thyme, rosemary, cinnamon, nutmeg, and cloves. Use herbs and spices generously in your dishes. They add depth and holiday flair without any added carbs, keeping your meal festive and flavorful.

Skip The Sugar, Keep The Sweet

- Desserts are a key part of Thanksgiving, and you don't have to miss out. Use natural Keto-approved sweeteners like stevia, erythritol, or monk fruit to create desserts that satisfy your sweet tooth without spiking your blood sugar. Look for recipes like pumpkin pie with an almond flour crust or pecan bars with a low-carb twist.

Watch out for Hidden Carbs

- Holiday recipes often contain hidden carbs in sauces, gravies, and marinades. Opt for homemade versions whenever possible, so you control the ingredients. Use broth or cream-based sauces instead of flour-thickened ones, and avoid recipes with added sugars.

Limit Alcohol or Choose Wisely

- If you plan to drink, stick to low-carb options like dry wines or spirits (gin, vodka, whiskey) with soda water or sparkling water as mixers. Be mindful of mixers that contain hidden sugars, as they can quickly add up.

Stay Hydrated and Snack Smart!

- Sometimes we confuse thirst with hunger. Make sure to drink plenty of water throughout the day, especially if you're also enjoying a cocktail or two. Have a few Keto-friendly snacks, like nuts, cheese, or deviled eggs, on hand before the main meal to help manage your hunger and avoid overindulging later.

Slow Down and Savor!

- Eating slowly and enjoying each bite can help you feel more satisfied. Remember, the holidays are about connection, gratitude, and creating memories. Take time to enjoy the moment, appreciate your food, and connect with loved ones.

Focus On Gratitude – Not Just The Food!

- Thanksgiving is about much more than the meal. Take a moment to reflect on what you're grateful for—your health, your journey, and the support of family and friends. Staying in a positive, grateful mindset can make it easier to enjoy the day without feeling restricted or deprived.

With the help of the Virta community, I was able to lose a significant amount of inflammation, which directly led to noticeable weight loss. This community became my lifeline, providing accountability and constant encouragement on my ketogenic journey. From sharing delicious, low-carb recipes to offering practical tips and tricks, the Virta community was there every step of the way. Together, we tackled meal planning, managed cravings, and celebrated each success. The support I received truly made the ketogenic lifestyle easier and more enjoyable, helping me achieve sustainable health and weight-loss results.

Finding Virta online was a game-changer! Their straightforward application process makes it easy to start, and many insurance plans now cover Virta's services, making this powerful support system accessible to many people. Once you're in, Virta equips you with all the essentials for a successful journey: a high-quality weight scale, a food scale, and tools to track blood glucose and ketone levels. They also provide books filled with recipes, practical guidelines, and valuable tips to help you stay on track. With Virta, you're fully supported and ready to dive into your health goals with confidence!

T u r k e y

This Keto-friendly turkey recipe is infused with fresh herbs, butter, and garlic, making it tender, juicy, and full of holiday flavor without the need for sugary marinades or carb-heavy ingredients. This recipe will yield a delicious main course that keeps you and your guests coming back for more.

Ingredients:

- 1 whole turkey (10-12 pounds), thawed if frozen
- 1/2 cup unsalted butter, softened
- 4 cloves garlic, minced
- 2 tbsp rosemary
- 2 tbsp thyme
- 2 tbsp sage
- 1 tbsp parsley
- 1 tbsp sea salt
- 1 tsp black pepper
- 1 lemon, halved
- 1 large onion, quartered
- 2 cups chicken or turkey broth, for basting

Instructions:

- Preheat your oven to 325°F (165°C).
- Pat the turkey dry with paper towels, both inside and out, to ensure the skin crisps up in the oven.
- Gently loosen the skin on the breast of the turkey by sliding your fingers under it, creating a pocket between the skin and meat.

- In a small bowl, mix the softened butter with minced garlic, chopped rosemary, thyme, sage, parsley, salt, and pepper.
- Carefully rub about 3/4 of the herb butter under the skin of the turkey breast, then rub the remaining butter all over the outside of the turkey, making sure it's evenly coated.

- Place the lemon halves and onion quarters inside the turkey cavity. This adds flavor and moisture without adding carbs.

- Place the turkey on a rack in a roasting pan, breast side up.
- Pour 1 cup of broth into the bottom of the pan.
- Cover the turkey loosely with aluminum foil and roast for about 2.5 to 3 hours (roughly 15 minutes per pound), basting with additional broth every 30 minutes to keep the turkey moist.

- For a golden, crispy skin, remove the foil during the last 30 minutes of cooking.
- Use a meat thermometer to check for doneness; the turkey is ready when the thickest part of the breast reaches 165°F (74°C) and the thighs reach 175°F (80°C).

- Remove the turkey from the oven, cover it with foil, and let it rest for 20-30 minutes before carving. This allows the juices to redistribute, keeping the meat tender and juicy.

- **Optional Gravy:** Use the pan drippings to make a Keto-friendly gravy. Simply add a bit of heavy cream and xanthan gum as a thickener instead of flour or cornstarch.
- **Extra Flavor Boost:** For even more flavor, add a few sprigs of fresh herbs and a garlic bulb, halved, to the bottom of the pan while roasting.

Enjoy a perfectly seasoned, low-carb turkey as the centerpiece of your Thanksgiving feast!

Nutritional Information:

- **Calories:** 320
- **Protein:** 45g
- **Fat:** 15g
  - **Saturated Fat:** 7g
- **Carbohydrates:** 1g

- - Fiber: 0g
  - Net Carbs: 1g
- **Sugars:** 0g
- **Sodium:** 350mg

Notes:

- **Protein** comes primarily from the turkey meat.
- **Fat** content is from the butter and turkey skin. If you use less butter, this amount will decrease slightly.
- **Carbs** are minimal, largely coming from the fresh herbs, which add a very small amount of carbs but pack in a lot of flavor.

This low-carb, high-protein turkey is ideal for Keto as it provides a satisfying main course with virtually no impact on carb intake, keeping you on track with your dietary goals this Thanksgiving!

Page Intentionally Left Blank

Keto Cornbread Dressing

Ingredients for Cornbread:

- 1 cup almond flour
- 2 tbsp coconut flour
- 1 tsp baking powder
- 1/4 tsp salt
- 2 large eggs
- 1/4 cup heavy cream
- 2 tbsp melted butter
- 1/2 tsp apple cider vinegar

Ingredients for Dressing:

- 1 batch of Keto Cornbread (from above), cubed and toasted
- 1 tbsp olive oil or butter
- 1/2 cup onion, finely chopped
- 1/2 cup celery, finely chopped
- 1/4 cup parsley
- 1 tbsp sage
- 1 tbsp rosemary
- 1 tbsp thyme
- 1/2 tsp salt
- 1/4 tsp black pepper
- 1/2 cup chicken or turkey broth, plus more as needed
- 1 large egg, beaten

Instructions :
Step 1 : Make the Keto Cornbread

1. Preheat oven to 350°F (175°C) and grease a small baking dish.
2. In a mixing bowl, combine almond flour, coconut flour, baking powder, and salt.
3. In another bowl, whisk together eggs, heavy cream, melted butter, and apple cider vinegar.
4. Pour the wet ingredients into the dry ingredients and mix until combined.

5. Pour the batter into the prepared baking dish and bake for 20-25 minutes or until golden and a toothpick inserted comes out clean.
6. Allow to cool, then cut into cubes and toast them on a baking sheet at 350°F (175°C) for 10 minutes until lightly crispy.

Step 2 : Prepare the Dressing

1. Preheat the oven to 350°F (175°C) again.
2. In a large skillet, heat the olive oil or butter over medium heat. Add the onion and celery and sauté until softened, about 5 minutes.
3. In a large bowl, combine the toasted cornbread cubes, sautéed onion and celery, parsley, sage, rosemary, thyme, salt, and pepper.
4. Pour the broth and beaten egg over the mixture and gently toss to combine. Add more broth if needed to reach your desired moisture level.
5. Transfer the mixture to a greased baking dish and bake for 25-30 minutes, until the dressing is golden brown on top and heated through.

Nutritional Information (per serving based on 8 servings)

- **Calories:** 190
- **Protein:** 6g
- **Fat:** 16g
    - **Saturated Fat:** 5g
- **Carbohydrates:** 6g
    - **Fiber:** 3g
    - **Net Carbs:** 3g
- **Sugars:** 1g
- **Sodium:** 300mg

Notes:

- **Net Carbs:** The 3g net carbs per serving make this dressing a great choice for those following a Keto lifestyle.
- **Moisture Level:** Keto cornbread tends to be more crumbly, so add extra broth if you prefer a softer, more traditional texture.
- **Fresh Herbs:** These give the dressing authentic holiday flavor. If using dried herbs, reduce the quantity by half.

Enjoy this delicious low-carb twist on a Thanksgiving classic, perfect for pairing with your herb-roasted turkey!

Page Intentionally Left Blank

Cauliflower Mashed "Potatoes"

This creamy, buttery cauliflower mash is the perfect low-carb alternative to traditional mashed potatoes. It's smooth, delicious, and pairs perfectly with any main dish, making it an ideal side for your Keto Thanksgiving feast.

Ingredients:

- 1 large head of cauliflower, cut into florets (about 6 cups)
- 3 tbsp unsalted butter
- 2 tbsp cream cheese, softened
- 1/4 cup heavy cream
- 1/2 tsp garlic powder
- Salt and pepper, to taste
- 2 tbsp chives (optional for garnish)

Instructions:

- **Steam Method:** Place the cauliflower florets in a steamer basket over a pot of boiling water. Cover and steam for 10-12 minutes, or until the cauliflower is very tender.
- **Boil Method:** Alternatively, you can boil the cauliflower florets in salted water for about 10 minutes, until fork-tender. Drain well.

Blend The Cauliflower:

- Transfer the cooked cauliflower to a food processor or high-powered blender. Add the butter, softened cream cheese, heavy cream, and garlic powder.
- Blend until smooth and creamy, scraping down the sides as needed. If the mixture is too thick, add a bit more heavy cream until you reach your desired consistency.

Season and Serve:

- Season the cauliflower mash with salt and pepper to taste.
- Transfer to a serving bowl and garnish with chopped fresh chives, if desired.

Nutrional Information: (per serving, based on 6 servings)

- **Calories:** 110
- **Protein:** 3g
- **Fat:** 9g
  - o **Saturated Fat:** 6g
- **Carbohydrates:** 6g
  - o **Fiber:** 3g
  - o **Net Carbs:** 3g
- **Sugars:** 3g
- **Sodium:** 100mg (varies based on added salt)

Tips:

- **Flavor Variations:** For extra flavor, try adding roasted garlic, grated Parmesan cheese, or a sprinkle of cheddar cheese before blending.
- **Texture:** For a chunkier mash, blend less and pulse a few times until you reach your desired consistency.
- **Reheating:** Cauliflower mash can be reheated gently on the stovetop or in the microwave. Add a splash of heavy cream or butter to keep it creamy.

Cauliflower Potato Salad

Ingredients:

This Keto-friendly cauliflower "potato" salad has all the classic flavors of traditional potato salad but without the carbs. Creamy, tangy, and loaded with flavor, it's the perfect side dish for any occasion.

Ingredients:

- 1 large head of cauliflower, cut into bite-sized florets (about 6 cups)
- 2 large hard-boiled eggs, chopped
- 1/4 cup mayonnaise
- 2 tbsp sour cream
- 1 tbsp Dijon mustard
- 1 tsp apple cider vinegar
- 1/4 cup celery, finely chopped
- 1/4 cup sugar free sweet gherkins, finely chopped
- 2 tbsp red onion, finely chopped
- 1 tbsp dill
- Salt and pepper, to taste
- Paprika, for garnish (optional)

Instructions:

Cook The Cauliflower:

- Bring a large pot of salted water to a boil. Add the cauliflower florets and cook for 5-7 minutes, until they're just tender but not mushy.
- Drain and let the cauliflower cool completely, then pat dry with paper towels to remove any excess moisture.

Prepare The Dressing:

- In a large mixing bowl, combine the mayonnaise, sour cream, Dijon mustard, and apple cider vinegar. Stir well to combine.

Assemble The Salad:

- Add the cooled cauliflower florets to the bowl with the dressing, along with the chopped eggs, celery, dill pickles, red onion, and fresh dill.
- Gently toss everything together until the cauliflower is well-coated in the dressing. Season with salt and pepper to taste.

Chill And Serve:

- Cover and refrigerate the salad for at least 1 hour to allow the flavors to meld.
- Before serving, sprinkle with a bit of paprika for color, if desired.

Nutritional Information (per serving, based on 6 servings)

- **Calories:** 140
- **Protein:** 3g
- **Fat:** 12g
  - **Saturated Fat:** 3g
- **Carbohydrates:** 5g
  - **Fiber:** 2g
  - **Net Carbs:** 3g
- **Sugars:** 1g
- **Sodium:** 150mg (varies based on added salt and pickles)

Tips:

- **Additions:** For more flavor, add 1-2 chopped green onions or a sprinkle of crumbled bacon.
- **Texture:** Make sure the cauliflower is fully cooled and patted dry to keep the salad creamy without extra moisture.
- **Storage:** This salad keeps well in the fridge for up to 3 days, making it an excellent make-ahead option.

Enjoy this delicious, Keto-friendly cauliflower "potato" salad as a side that's both creamy and satisfying, perfect for your low-carb lifestyle!

Page Intentionally Left Blank

This Keto-friendly green bean casserole skips the carb-heavy canned soups and fried onions, using fresh ingredients to create a creamy, flavorful dish with a crunchy topping. It's perfect for a holiday meal or any family dinner.

Ingredients: Green Beans & Sauce

- 1 lb fresh green beans, trimmed and cut into 1-inch pieces (about 4 cups)
- 2 tbsp butter
- 1/2 medium onion, finely chopped
- 2 cloves garlic, minced
- 1 cup mushrooms, sliced
- 1 cup heavy cream
- 1/2 cup chicken or vegetable broth
- 1/2 tsp Worcestershire sauce
- Salt and pepper, to taste

Crunchy Topping

- 1/2 cup pork rinds, crushed (for crunch)
- 1/4 cup grated Parmesan cheese
- 1/4 cup almond flour
- 1 tbsp butter, melted:

Instructions:

Prepare the Green Beans:

- Preheat oven to 350°F (175°C).
- Blanch the green beans by bringing a pot of salted water to a boil. Add the green beans and cook for 4-5 minutes until they're just tender. Drain and set aside.

Make The Creamy Sauce:

- In a large skillet, melt the butter over medium heat. Add the onion, garlic, and mushrooms, and cook until softened, about 5-6 minutes.
- Add the heavy cream, chicken broth, Worcestershire sauce, salt, and pepper. Bring the mixture to a simmer, stirring frequently. Let it cook for about 5-7 minutes, or until the sauce thickens slightly.
- Remove from heat, add the blanched green beans, and stir until the beans are well-coated in the sauce.

Prepare the Topping

- In a small bowl, combine the crushed pork rinds, Parmesan cheese, almond flour, and melted butter. Stir until well-mixed.

Assemble and Bake

- Pour the green bean mixture into a greased baking dish.
- Sprinkle the topping evenly over the green beans.
- Bake in the preheated oven for 20-25 minutes, until the topping is golden and the casserole is bubbling around the edges.

Nutritional Information (per serving, based on 6 servings)

- **Calories:** 220
- **Protein:** 6g
- **Fat:** 20g
  - **Saturated Fat:** 10g
- **Carbohydrates:** 6g
  - **Fiber:** 2g
  - **Net Carbs:** 4g
- **Sugars:** 2g
- **Sodium:** 180mg (varies with salt added)

Tips

- **Make Ahead:** Assemble the casserole (without the topping) up to 1 day in advance and refrigerate. Add the topping just before baking.
- **Topping Options:** If you don't have pork rinds, you can replace them with extra almond flour, although it may slightly alter the texture.
- **Mushroom Alternatives:** For a mushroom-free version, replace them with chopped zucchini or extra onions for flavor.

This Keto green bean casserole brings all the comforting flavors of the classic dish without the carbs, perfect for a holiday gathering!

Page Intentionally Left Blank

Cauliflower Mac & Cheese

This creamy, cheesy, and Keto-friendly cauliflower "mac" and cheese is a fantastic low-carb alternative to the traditional dish. It features tender cauliflower in a rich cheese sauce that's sure to satisfy your comfort food cravings.

Ingredients

- 1 large head of cauliflower, cut into bite-sized florets (about 6 cups)
- 1 cup heavy cream
- 2 cups shredded sharp cheddar cheese
- 1/2 cup shredded mozzarella cheese
- 1/4 cup cream cheese, softened
- 1/4 tsp garlic powder
- 1/4 tsp onion powder
- Salt and pepper, to taste
- 1/4 cup grated Parmesan cheese
- 1/4 cup pork rinds, crushed (for optional crunchy topping)

Instructions:

Prepare the Cauliflower:

- Preheat oven to 375°F (190°C).
- Bring a large pot of salted water to a boil. Add the cauliflower florets and cook for 5-7 minutes, until just tender. Drain well and set aside.

Make the Cheese Sauce

- In a medium saucepan over medium heat, combine the heavy cream and cream cheese, stirring until the cream cheese melts and the mixture is smooth.
- Add the shredded cheddar and mozzarella cheese gradually, stirring constantly until melted and smooth.
- Stir in the garlic powder, onion powder, salt, and pepper to taste.

Combine

- Place the cooked cauliflower florets in a baking dish. Pour the cheese sauce over the cauliflower and stir gently to coat.
- Sprinkle the grated Parmesan on top. If you like a crunchy topping, sprinkle the crushed pork rinds over the top as well.

Bake

- Bake in the preheated oven for 20-25 minutes, until the top is bubbly and golden brown.

Nutritional Information (per serving, based on 6 servings)

- **Calories:** 290
- **Protein:** 11g
- **Fat:** 25g
  - **Saturated Fat:** 14g
- **Carbohydrates:** 6g
  - **Fiber:** 2g
  - **Net Carbs:** 4g
- **Sugars:** 2g
- **Sodium:** 400mg (varies based on added salt and cheese)

Tips

- **Cheese Options:** Feel free to use other Keto-friendly cheeses like Gouda, Monterey Jack, or Gruyere for different flavors.
- **Make Ahead:** You can assemble the dish ahead of time, cover, and refrigerate. Bake just before serving.
- **Extra Flavor:** Add a pinch of smoked paprika or cayenne pepper to the cheese sauce for a bit of extra kick.

This Keto cauliflower mac and cheese is creamy, satisfying, and packed with cheesy goodness, making it the perfect comfort food without the carbs!

Page Intentionally Left Blank

Keto Turkey Gravy

This rich, flavorful Keto turkey gravy is thickened with xanthan gum instead of flour, keeping it low in carbs but full of savory flavor. It's the perfect accompaniment to your holiday turkey and is ready in just a few minutes!

Ingredients:

- 2 cups turkey drippings or turkey broth (or a combination of both)
- 2 tbsp unsalted butter
- 1/4 tsp xanthan gum (or up to 1/2 tsp for a thicker gravy)
- Salt and pepper, to taste
- 1/4 tsp garlic powder (optional)
- 1/4 tsp onion powder (optional)
- 1 tsp thyme or rosemary for extra flavor)

Instructions:

Heat the Drippings.

- In a medium saucepan over medium heat, melt the butter. Add the turkey drippings or broth and bring to a gentle simmer.

Thicken with Xanthan Gum:

- Gradually sprinkle in the xanthan gum, whisking continuously to avoid clumping. Start with 1/4 tsp, then add more if needed to reach your desired thickness.
- Continue whisking for 3-5 minutes as the gravy thickens. If it becomes too thick, add a little more broth or drippings to thin it out.

Season and Serve:

- Season the gravy with salt and pepper to taste. Add garlic powder, onion powder, and fresh herbs if desired.

- Serve warm over turkey, mashed cauliflower, or any other Keto-friendly side.

Nutritional Information (per ¼ cup serving, based on 8 servings)

- **Calories:** 40
- **Protein:** 1g
- **Fat:** 4g
  - **Saturated Fat:** 2g
- **Carbohydrates:** 0.5g
  - **Fiber:** 0g
  - **Net Carbs:** 0.5g
- **Sugars:** 0g
- **Sodium:** 200mg (varies based on broth and added salt)

Tips:

- **Adjusting Thickness:** Start with a small amount of xanthan gum, as a little goes a long way. You can always add more if needed.
- **Flavor Boosters:** If you like, add a splash of heavy cream for a richer gravy or a dash of Worcestershire sauce for extra depth.
- **Make Ahead:** This gravy can be made a day ahead and reheated on the stovetop. Just whisk to restore smoothness before serving.

Cheesy Broccoli & Cauliflower

Ingredients:

- 1 (12 or 16 oz) package of frozen broccoli florets
- 1 (12 oz) package cauliflower rice
- 1 small onion, finely diced
- 1 1/4 cups cream of mushroom soup
- 1/2 cup heavy cream
- 1 teaspoon salt
- 1/2 teaspoon black pepper
- 1/4 teaspoon garlic powder
- 1/4 teaspoon paprika
- 4 cups shredded mild or medium cheddar cheese
- Crushed pork rinds, for topping

Instructions:

1. Thaw the broccoli and cauliflower rice, then warm the broccoli in the microwave for 3-4 minutes. Drain any excess liquid, and cut the broccoli florets into bite-sized pieces.
2. Preheat your oven to 350°F. In a large mixing bowl, combine the warmed cauliflower rice, broccoli, diced onion, cream of mushroom soup, heavy cream, salt, pepper, garlic powder, paprika, and 1 1/2 to 2 cups of shredded cheddar cheese. Stir until all ingredients are thoroughly mixed.
3. Lightly spray a 9x13-inch baking dish (or two 8x8 pans) with avocado oil. Pour the mixture into the prepared dish, spreading it evenly. Sprinkle the remaining shredded cheddar cheese on top.
4. Bake at 350°F for 35-40 minutes if using a large dish, or 25-30 minutes for smaller dishes, until
5. the casserole is bubbly and the cheese begins to brown.
6. In the last 5 minutes of baking, sprinkle crushed pork rinds over the top for added crunch.
7. Let cool slightly before serving. This casserole also freezes well, so save leftovers for an easy, delicious meal later on!

Nutritional Information (per serving)

- **Calories:** 310
- **Fat:** 25g
- **Saturated Fat:** 15g
- **Cholesterol:** 70mg
- **Sodium:** 600mg
- **Carbohydrates:** 6gFiber: 2g
- **Net Carbs:** 4g
- **Protein:** 12g

Keto Pecan Pie

This Keto pecan pie has a deliciously buttery crust and a gooey, caramel-like filling, all while keeping carbs low and flavors high. It's the perfect dessert for any holiday table!

Ingredients:

Crust:

- 1 1/2 cups almond flour
- 1/4 cup coconut flour
- 1/4 cup powdered erythritol or monk fruit sweetener
- 1/4 tsp salt
- 1/4 cup unsalted butter, melted
- 1 large egg, beaten

Filling:

- 1 cup pecans, roughly chopped
- 1/2 cup unsalted butter
- 1/2 cup powdered erythritol or monk fruit sweetener
- 1/2 cup sugar-free maple syrup
- 3 large eggs
- 1 tsp vanilla extract
- 1/4 tsp salt

Instructions:

Prepare The Crust:

- Preheat the oven to 350°F (175°C). Grease a 9-inch pie dish.
- In a mixing bowl, combine the almond flour, coconut flour, powdered sweetener, and salt.
- Stir in the melted butter and beaten egg until a dough forms.
- Press the dough evenly into the bottom and up the sides of the prepared pie dish. Use a fork to poke a few holes in the crust to prevent bubbling.
- Bake the crust for 10-12 minutes, or until lightly golden. Remove from the oven and set aside.

Make The Filling:

- In a saucepan over medium heat, melt the butter and powdered sweetener together, stirring until the sweetener dissolves.
- Add the sugar-free maple syrup and cook for 2-3 minutes, stirring constantly until the mixture thickens slightly. Remove from heat and let cool for a few minutes.
- In a separate bowl, whisk the eggs, vanilla extract, and salt. Slowly whisk in the cooled butter mixture until well combined.
- Add the chopped pecans and stir to combine.

Assemble and Bake:

- Pour the pecan filling into the pre-baked crust, spreading it evenly.
- Bake for 35-40 minutes, until the filling is set and the pie is golden brown. The center should jiggle slightly when shaken.
- Remove from the oven and let cool completely before slicing. The filling will firm up as it cools.

Nutritional Information (per slice, based on 10 servings)

- **Calories:** 290
- **Protein:** 5g
- **Fat:** 28g
  - **Saturated Fat:** 8g
- **Carbohydrates:** 7g
  - **Fiber:** 4g
  - **Net Carbs:** 3g
- **Sugars:** 1g
- **Sodium:** 100mg

Tips:

- **Make Ahead:** This pie can be made the day before and stored in the refrigerator.
- **Serve with Whipped Cream:** A dollop of sugar-free whipped cream adds an extra touch of decadence!
- **Cooling Time:** Let the pie cool completely to ensure the filling firms up.

Enjoy this indulgent, Keto-friendly pecan pie that's both delicious and low in carbs!

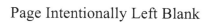
Page Intentionally Left Blank

Keto Pumpkin Pie

This Keto pumpkin pie delivers all the warm, spiced flavors of the traditional Thanksgiving favorite without the carbs. With a buttery almond flour crust and creamy pumpkin filling, it's the perfect ending to any holiday meal.

Ingredients:

- 1 1/2 cups almond flour
- 1/4 cup coconut flour
- 1/4 cup powdered erythritol or monk fruit sweetener
- 1/4 tsp salt
- 1/4 cup unsalted butter, melted
- 1 large egg, beaten

Filling:

- 1 cup canned pumpkin puree (not pumpkin pie filling)
- 2/3 cup heavy cream
- 1/2 cup powdered erythritol or monk fruit sweetener
- 2 large eggs
- 1 tsp vanilla extract
- 1 1/2 tsp ground cinnamon
- 1/2 tsp ground ginger
- 1/4 tsp ground nutmeg
- 1/4 tsp ground cloves
- 1/4 tsp salt

Instructions:

Prepare The Crust:

- Preheat oven to 350°F (175°C). Grease a 9-inch pie dish.
- In a mixing bowl, combine almond flour, coconut flour, powdered sweetener, and salt.
- Stir in the melted butter and beaten egg until a dough forms.

- Press the dough evenly into the bottom and up the sides of the pie dish. Use a fork to poke a few holes in the crust to prevent bubbling.
- Bake the crust for 10-12 minutes, or until lightly golden. Set aside to cool slightly.

Make The Filling:

- In a mixing bowl, whisk together the pumpkin puree, heavy cream, powdered sweetener, eggs, vanilla extract, cinnamon, ginger, nutmeg, cloves, and salt until smooth and well combined.

Assemble and Bake:

- Pour the pumpkin filling into the pre-baked crust, spreading it evenly.
- Bake for 40-50 minutes, or until the filling is set but still slightly jiggly in the center. If the crust starts to brown too much, cover the edges with foil.
- Remove from the oven and allow the pie to cool completely. The filling will continue to firm as it cools.

Nutritional Information (per slice, based on 10 servings)

- **Calories:** 180
- **Protein:** 4g
- **Fat:** 16g
  - **Saturated Fat:** 6g
- **Carbohydrates:** 7g
  - **Fiber:** 3g
  - **Net Carbs:** 4g
- **Sugars:** 2g
- **Sodium:** 80mg

Tips:

- **Chill Before Serving:** For best results, chill the pie for at least 1-2 hours before serving. This helps the filling set and makes it easier to slice.
- **Serve with Keto Whipped Cream:** A dollop of sugar-free whipped cream adds the perfect finishing touch.
- **Storage:** Store leftovers covered in the refrigerator for up to 3 days.

Enjoy this Keto pumpkin pie with all the classic flavor and none of the carbs! It's a delicious, low-carb way to celebrate the holidays.

Page Intentionally Left Blank

Conclusion

As we wrap up *Karbvelous Keto: Transform Your Plate, Transform Your Life - Thanksgiving Edition*, I hope you've found inspiration, flavor, and a renewed sense of possibility for your holiday meals. Living a Keto lifestyle, especially during the holidays, doesn't mean sacrificing the flavors, textures, and warmth that make Thanksgiving special. With the right recipes and a bit of planning, you can create a celebration that's both delicious and supportive of your health goals.

Thanksgiving is a time for connection, gratitude, and savoring life's blessings. Each recipe in this book was crafted to bring you a little closer to that feeling of gratitude—with dishes that help you stay true to your health journey without compromising on enjoyment. My wish for you is that this Thanksgiving will be memorable not just for the food, but for the joy of knowing you can indulge in holiday traditions while staying on track.

As you gather around the table with loved ones, may this feast remind you that you are capable of nourishing yourself with intention, of finding joy in food that fuels, and of celebrating your journey toward a healthier, happier you. Here's to a season full of health, happiness, and gratitude. Thank you for allowing *Karbvelous Keto* to be a part of your Thanksgiving celebration.

A b o u t   t h e   A u t h o r

Carolyn Boheler's journey with weight and health challenges began in 1987 when she was diagnosed with Hashimoto's disease. This autoimmune condition led to the destruction of her thyroid gland through radiation, causing her to struggle with weight issues for many years. However, Carolyn found hope and success through the ketogenic lifestyle. By embracing keto, she not only managed to lose the weight but also kept it off, transforming her life in the process.

In her new book, Carolyn shares the recipes and "tricks" that have made this lifestyle sustainable and achievable. Her personal experience and practical advice offer readers a blueprint for a healthier, more fulfilling life, making the journey not just possible but enjoyable.

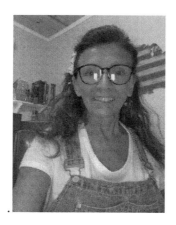

www.GoodSensePublishing.com

Karbvelous Keto

Transform Your Plate, Transform Your Life

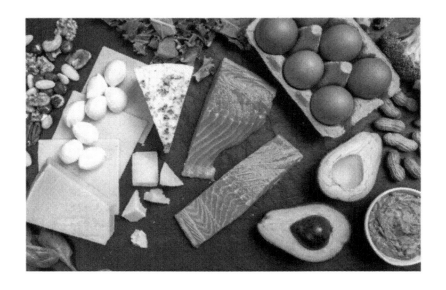

by: Carolyn Boheler, PhD

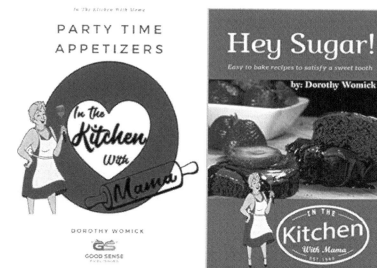

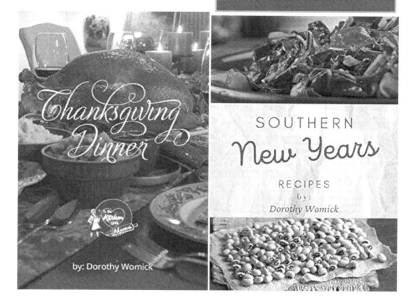

Available online at https://GoodSensePublishing.com

Acknowledgments

This book would not have been possible without the support and encouragement of many people. First and foremost, I want to thank my family and friends for their unwavering belief in me, even when the journey seemed long and difficult. Your love and support have been my greatest motivation.

To my medical team, thank you for your guidance and care over the years. Your expertise helped me navigate the challenges of Hashimoto's disease, and I am deeply grateful for your dedication to my health and well-being.

I also want to express my gratitude to the community, both online and offline, for sharing their experiences, tips, and encouragement. You have shown me that I am not alone on this journey, and your stories have inspired me to keep going.

A special thank you to my readers—your interest in this book is what drives me to share my story and my recipes. I hope that what I've learned and created will help you find success and joy in your keto journey.

Finally, to everyone who has contributed to this book, whether through feedback, taste-testing, or simply cheering me on—thank you. This book is a reflection of the love, support, and knowledge that I have been fortunate to receive, and I am honored to share it with all of you.

Please take the time to leave a review if you've enjoyed my books.

https://amzn.to/48ECEb6

Thank you so much!

I've included links to items found on Amazon that are used in the recipes within this book. When you click one of these links, I may earn a small commission, but rest assured, your price will not be higher because of it. Occasionally, you might even find a better deal!
The links are clickable on the Kindle or ebook versions, or you can find a page of links at www.GoodSensePublishing.

Made in the USA
Columbia, SC
23 November 2024

46998635R00028